WEIGHT LOSS SURGERY, A PATIENT'S PERSPECTIVE!

Information & insight the professionals don't have or can't relate to!

Arlanda Archible

WEIGHT LOSS SURGERY,
A PATIENT'S PERSPECTIVE!

© 2014 by Arlanda Archible

This book is not intended as a substitute for the medical advice of physicians.

The reader should regularly consult a physician in matters relating to his/her health and particularly with respect to any symptoms that may require diagnosis or medical attention.

No part of this book may be reproduced or transmitted in any form with the intention of reselling or distributing such copies without written permission from the publisher, except for brief quotations included in a review.

Published by: Arlanda Archible
                   Elk Grove, California
                   arlandarchible@outlook.com

First Printing, 2014
Printed in the United State of America
ISBN: 978-1-5007363-0-9

(All rights reserved)

Contents

Acknowledgements 4
Introduction 5
Chapter 1 – What Should I Do 11
Chapter 2 - Frequently Asked Questions 15
Chapter 3 – The Decision 21
Chapter 4 – The Journey 27
Chapter 6 – What The @#$%^ Did I Just Do? 39
Chapter 7 – The Mourning 45
Chapter 8 – The Reactions 52
Chapter 9 – Processing the Anger 58
Chapter 10 –The Loss 64
Chapter 11 –The Fear of Regaining The weight 81
Chapter 12 – The Faith in yourself, your decisions, and in God 87
Your Chapter – Make Peace with Your Decision 91
Your Beginning – Never the End! 93

Acknowledgements

I am so grateful for these folk, no really I am☺

You know I didn't do this alone, so let's get the customary thanks out of the way.

I thank God, my Lord and Savior Jesus Christ for keeping and teaching me.

I thank my family for: holding my hand, listening to my mouth, enduring the peaks & valleys, and supporting this dream.

My honey, perfectly abnormal husband, George, my favorite child (and only one) my baby- Desiree (Dezi-Boo), My Rock, My 911, My free therapist- Shawana, Reality Check Couple-Lady & Steve, Fun Monitor-Wanda, Reliable-Silent Support - Twinkle, Wisdom-Other Dad- Luther (paw paw), Partner in Crime, work husband, all around cool guy -Greg, My Lovely Ladies: Tenise, Pele, Veronica, Lakeeta, Delisa, Tommie, Tina, Tohana, Sharyl, Holly, Danelle, Lisa, Sharon, Maureen, Nina, Jessica, Rhanika, Rochelle, Deshawn, Karmalita, Dimitra, Gaynelle, Audrey, Aunt Martha, Weight monitor -Aunt Arcille, My giggle-snort-laugh guy; Darren (Qubby), my adopted kids-youth-inspiration (Aaron, Porsche, Kareena, Tatiana, Sharonda, Theresa, Terell, Zanyell). The completion expert- Mike Rounds, Mother Lula & SSCC intercessory prayer team, Bishop Bob Jackson, Bishop Simmons, Pastor Dr. D Simmons, Minister Daniel Easter, Pastor and First Lady Washington

Introduction

Ok folks, put on your seatbelts *(extender belts available upon request☺)* and let's get honest, real, and raw about weight loss surgery (WLS).

No, I am not a medical professional nor am I in the medical field, but I invite you to look into the joy and pain of weight loss surgery with me.

You may ask yourself, ok why should I believe or even consider what you have to say about WLS?

I don't blame you one bit, but ask yourself this question:

When considering a new restaurant, or if you should check out a new movie, do you value the opinion of someone who has already eaten at the restaurant or has gone to see the movie?

I suspect that you'd especially value the opinion if that someone is just like you, not a chef or a movie producer.

So the answer is: YES, of course you would listen to them!

So when it comes to listening to somebody about WLS, I'm the *"go-to person"* because I had weight loss surgery in 2007 and I promise to be candid and embarrassingly open about this voyage.

I promise to bare all and share all of my honest opinions, manic research and experiences; good, bad, funny, and ugly.

Up for discussion are topics such as:

- Is this selfish?
- What type of surgery should or shouldn't be considered?
- What to expect?
- Who to trust?
- Why do people keep saying I've changed?

Also, what to do *after* making the big decision?

And by decision, I also mean deciding NOT to proceed with WLS.

To make this book easier to read and understand, I've broken the material down into the things that I experienced.

They might not make logical sense to an English teacher, but they make sense to anyone who's even thinking about WLS as a solution to their weight concerns.

So what is weight loss surgery anyway?

In its simplest form, (or so I thought), weight loss surgery (WLS) is a tool to lose weight utilizing medical intervention.

Many use the blanket term "weight loss surgery" because there are so many methods and processes one can chose from, and WLS seems to cover the gamut.

So let's see how it works:

1. One gets wheeled into an operating room in a slightly to morbidly obese drugged up state
2. The minutes and hours tick by, and
3. The 'magic' happens.

Next thing you know, the patient's internal organs have been: severed, altered, removed, and/or added to and instantly the patient begins to lose weight.

Voila, it's a wrap, sounds like a plan to me! An easy fix - a solid solution, a means to an end, but perhaps not.

I found out that it's a bit more involved than the afore mentioned 1, 2, 3 method so please never allow someone to tell you it's an easy out.

There is nothing *easy* about the decision, up to and including, the long-term maintenance and after care.

WLS is a tool, similar to other medical interventions.

Anyone can learn how to eat smaller or liquid portions, or alter eating behavior *(a short term solution for me mostly☺)* but what about thinking smaller?

- But what about missing the satisfaction of an adult sized bacon cheeseburger, and its juices dripping down your wrist?

- What about learning to deal with the people (well-meaning and all) who are monitoring your weight loss, weight gain, and every morsel of food that enters your mouth?

- What about the new attention and looks one gets once the weight drops off, and the anger one feels about *not* getting the attention before?

- What about the constant fear of gaining the weight back and the impending outcome of pulling the fat suit back on, as it were?

Yeah guys, what about all of that?

All of these are valid and real thoughts that enter the minds of those who consider or undergo WLS.

You are NOT alone!

One final note, I really like quotes... short ones, long ones, funny and spiritual.

So I am just letting you know they will be sprinkled throughout, just like raisins in a quality carrot cake. ENJOY!

Attention Weight Loss Shoppers!

Please pay attention because this part is important!

It's a Road Map to this little book.

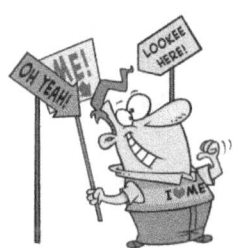

*"Never let outside voices speak louder than **your** inner voice."* –S. Thomas

You have permission to check out the headings of each chapter and feel free to skip around to skim and read the chapter or process you are currently going through or interested in!

There is NO need to go in order... dog-ear, highlight, bookmark, and e-save, add a sticky note and read from the final chapter forward!

It doesn't matter how you do it, but know there is something in here that will help you along the way.

My sole purpose for writing this book was to let potential and current WLS patients know they aren't alone, and there is someone who can relate to their situation.

In fact, I dare say I was *compelled* to share my journey for I knew someone *would* benefit.

Please use the blank sections provided at the end of each chapter as a section for notes, primary journal, supplementary journal, or doodle space.

OK, Take A Deep Breath... Let's Start!

Chapter 1 – What Should I Do

When contemplating weight loss surgery (WLS) I wanted someone I could relate to, cry with, vent to, and chat with.

I wanted a diet buddy and someone with me while I suffered and enjoyed my journey.

In fact I wanted a buddy not only to discuss things with along the way, but heck I wanted somebody to go through every aspect of WLS **with** me *(before, during, and after surgery).*

I knew I had to trust this person implicitly and know they weren't judging or laughing at me, and had no ulterior motives,.

Well I didn't have that ONE person per se, but I had a few individuals who loved and listened to me. Most of all I relied on my faith and relationship with God to see me through the process.

I am writing this book so that **you** have a pal to go through the process with YOU. Please read the book as you proceed on your journey, I will be the girlfriend and confidant you desire and crave.

Each chapter may not mirror your exact challenge or stage, but most emotions and challenges will be addressed.

I know for sure, I experienced more mood-swings than a person with multiple personality disorder (no really, I did), so I am certain most issues will be covered.

There are **three** ways one can approach any life changing decision, especially one as life altering as WLS:

1. Research and make an informed decision

2. Commit instantly and never look back, and lastly

3. Proceed with trepidation and urgency due to lack of options, (because circumstances mandate an immediate action).

Let's check them all out.

For the **first** approach, one may choose to proceed armed with: data, caution, *and* trepidation. I mean basically research and study!

We are fortunate to live in a media rich age, which can be a blessing as well as a curse.

Being over informed and taking in every bit and blog out there can cause sensory overload.

However, do become informed about the subject, and *weigh* (horrible pun intended) your options cautiously to make the best choice.

When proceeding with "trepidation," I mean simply, even though you are scared out of your wits, press on toward a decision, even if WLS is not for you.

The **second** approach is, jump in head-first! Just make a decision, commit and do what your heart and head says is best, and then jump!

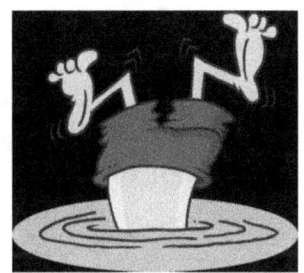

The **third** option is to be told that you really don't have a decision to make other than lose weight or die.

In essence your physician *tells (the medical community says suggests)* you this is a path you should and must take to survive.

The most difficult approach I and most people take is: combine them all and seal the deal by allowing your moral compass to guide you to the finish line.

I used one final decision making tool, prayer.

This worked (and still does) for me. I considered all of the possible outcomes and allowed the Lord to guide me on the right path.

You may use other tools, but never believe you are out of options.

There is no definite right way to make a "big" decision.

Even if you cross your T's and dot your I's and read everything out there about WLS, you may still be left with doubt, and questions.

Any kind of life changing decision should be taken seriously and given an appropriate amount of time and consideration.

IT'S OK, TAKE YOUR TIME.

The goal of this book is NOT to help you make the decision, NOT to inform you, and NOT to scare you.

I am not a physician, nutritionist, psychologist, counselor, or clergy.

However, I am Christian woman who embarked on the journey and would like to share with you, ***What The Professionals Don't Tell You About weight Loss Surgery!***

Chapter 2 - Frequently Asked Questions

It's interesting that as soon as people find out that I've undergone WLS, they ask me a whole bunch of questions about WLS and my experience so I thought it would make sense if I share what other people's concerns are *(and I'll bet they're yours too☺)* about WLS.

Q: Which WLS surgery did you have, and what type of surgery would you recommend?

A: I had the gastric-bypass, Roux-en-Y procedure. The types of surgeries are as varied as the physicians that administer them. As for a recommendation, only a health professional can tell you which procedure is the best fit for you. And for goodness sakes, please check out the physician. (Including how many surgeries they have performed.)

Q: Did the surgery hurt?

A: Yeah it hurts – it's surgery and they cut you with a knife! Yeech! But honestly, the recovery was not difficult or lengthy. Childbirth and knee surgery hurt far worse, and caused more discomfort during the recovery process.

Q: **How much will I lose?**

A: The short answer is, it varies. I went from 310 lbs. to 170 lbs.

Q: **How long does it take for the weight to come off?**

A: Regardless of the type of surgery, a year is the rule of thumb

Q: **What things will I have to do for the rest of my life, if I get WLS?**

A: Take vitamins; be aware of what and how much you eat, and follow the healthcare rules for life. An example of one of the rules is: *always choose water over other beverages.*

Q: **What about all of the excess skin and/or follow up surgery?**

A: I am 7 years post WLS, and I have yet to surgically remove the excess skin. Quality foundation garments are my friends! Some WLS programs include cosmetic surgery aftercare, but my health coverage did not.

Q: **Is hair loss a real concern?**

A: I did experience hair loss, in fact most people who lose weight rapidly, via WLS or diet and exercise, experience hair loss. I am blessed to have more hair than your average bear, so even with the loss my hair was never visibly thin. The market is flooded and full of products-tricks-and-tips to minimize and camouflage hair loss.

Q: **Are the psychiatric evaluation or pre-therapy appointments helpful?**

A: During my pre WLS prep phase, I would have answered HECK NO. In retrospect, I say yes 100%. Talk to a professional, ask questions, and dig deep. The mental "prep work" is one of the most important factors of post WLS success.

Q: **Were you able to eat some of your favorite foods after WLS?**

A: Before WLS, a fried egg sandwich was my go to pleasure snack. Post WLS, my desire and tolerance for such "semi-rich" snack food is ZERO. But some of my favs I am still able to enjoy on occasion and in smaller quantities.

Q: **Is exercise as important as the healthcare pros suggest, and will it become easier?**

A: Exercise is important, but honestly, I do not do as much as I should or as little as I used to. Exercise is more than just moving your body; it gets you in the mind frame and habits of a healthier lifestyle.

Q: ***What are some of the benefits of WLS that may not be mentioned in healthcare literature?***

A: I experienced an improved sex life, clearer skin, less sinus congestion, and I no longer fear plane or arena seats. In short, little *"challenges or annoyances you endure"* that you may not associate with being overweight are probably indeed impacted by excess weight in some way.

Q: ***Does dumping syndrome occur often?***

A: In most instances, dumping is caused by wrong choices. In my case, it lessened with time, and was so uncomfortable I STILL avoid those things which caused it in the first place.

Q: ***Did you use, or do you suggest a support group?***

A: There were group classes mandated by my healthcare provider, so I did attend some sessions. Honestly I used this journal, turned book, for my primary support group. But, know that a laptop can't: share experiences, triumphs, tragedies, and can't talk back. So a support group is definitely a good idea.

Q: What about getting pregnant or fertility related issues after WLS.

A: Since I am not a health professional, I cannot answer with specifics. I will however say, MANY post WLS women gain about 20+ pounds for 9 months after losing weight! Some male post WLS spouses gain the same amount for 9 months. So you do the math.

Q: Was there a period of depression?

A: There was more depression for me after WLS than before surgery; I later learned this was not uncommon. However, I gained an appreciation for improved health and mobility which helped balance the negative thoughts.

Q: Do you regret having WLS?

A: For me, it was the absolute right decision. So, nah.

Your thoughts, questions, concerns, or notes:

Chapter 3 – The Decision

"Trust that still, small, constant whisper. Trust the constant tug. Trust yourself. God whispers and the world is loud, often the whisper knows what your head has yet to figure out." -Me

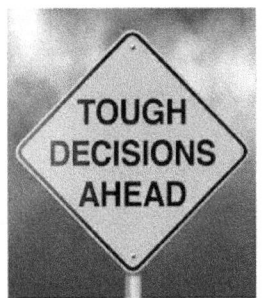

Deciding to consider weight loss surgery (WLS) exposes one to a mind-field of questions, doubts, and self-exploration and guess what, that is ok!

No sane individual can or should effectively consider weight loss surgery, or even decide which surgery to have without thinking twice.

The reasons to consider having weight loss surgery are as varied as the procedures themselves.

We won't even discuss the varied outcomes of the different procedures. I thought surgery was the easier way to reach my weight loss goal (it is definitely not).

Many friends and relatives viewed WLS as an easier choice as well.

Allow me to validate your concerns; WLS may be viewed as easy, but it is anything but!

Being a single parent, I thought to myself how dare I risk my life and possibly leave my child without a mother, just to lose weight?

Was I being incredibly selfish?

Was my lack of self-control that pathetic?

Although my WLS was precipitated by failing arthritic knees, I thought to myself (as many have admittedly thought as well) is there a part of me that just wants to look better? Am I doing this for the right reasons?

If I feel better, and the knee pain lessens is that just the icing on the cake?

Seriously, if WLS was any other type of surgery that would simultaneously enhance our health and appearance, would it be considered as taboo? I think not!!!

Often times we find it **easy** to make decisions for our loved ones, such as children or family members.

Decisions such as: what medicine to give them, which schools should they attend, what is best for them to eat, what time they should return from the school dance?

But when it comes to ourselves (breathe in deeply), we often hesitate with ambivalence and indecision.

Sometimes we should turn on *mommy-wife-employee-volunteer-superhero mode* FOR OURSELVES.

How will you best serve and love the ones you care for if you are not operating at optimal level?

Optimal for you may not mean WLS, but do make it part of the decision making process.

We are all familiar with the *"emergency oxygen mask analogy,"* but I will give it anyway.

When on a plane, the flight attendant instructs parents to place the oxygen mask on themselves first before placing the mask on the child.

In short, if mom or dad is not awake, they can't help the child.

Deciding to have WLS is a very similar decision.

Oddly the hardest part of my decision making process was feeling guilty about taking so long to decide.

I heard co-workers and friends of friends talk about how resolute they were in making the decision to have surgery.

In fact, I sought advice from a co-worker who had the surgery and was told that I was stupid for even thinking about it twice.

"What are you waiting for?" she exclaimed.

I thought to myself, why should I be in such a quandary?

Certainly the decision was easy enough for her.

WELL THAT IS CRAZY!

Take the amount of time that is right for YOU.

Surely all of the doctors suggesting the surgery can't be wrong, those stoic all-knowing men and women of the medical profession urging you to hurry and get it done, you will be whole.

No one knows you like you, just rest in that knowledge.

The important thing to know is, the decision to proceed or not to proceed with WLS is as personal as it gets.

This decision should be mulled over with all of the intensity of a child considering a plate full of cauliflower at dinnertime.

If you have done the introspective work and decided WLS is not for you, then rest knowing you have valued and loved yourself enough to have considered the option.

Find peace with your decision and revisit the subject when and if the time is right, and you will know when the time is right.

For once, this is about you.

Yes, you may desire to lose weight in the end to be able to play with your children more, get off of meds, heck to be able to get off of the couch, find a spouse, or even get on an airplane.

But, this begins and ends with YOU. So, if others don't agree with you, too bad.

"You have to decide what your highest priorities are and have the courage – pleasantly, smilingly, non-apologetically – to say 'no' to other things. And the way to do that is by having a bigger 'yes' burning inside." – Stephen Covey.

Decision by definition is: *"a choice that you make about something after thinking about it; the result of deciding."*

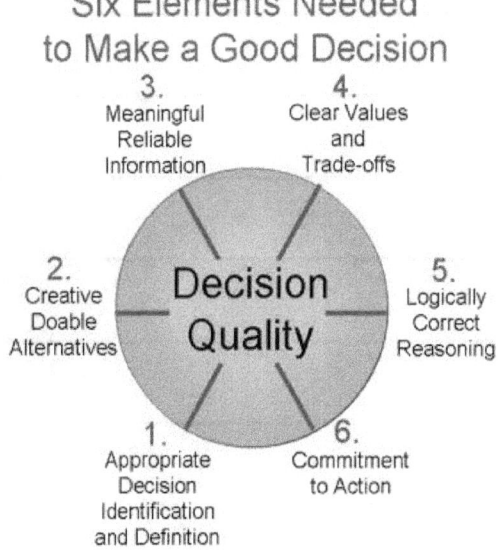

Your thoughts, questions, concerns, or notes:

Chapter 4 – The Journey

"To get through the hardest journey we need take only one step at a time, but we must keep on stepping."
– Chinese Proverb

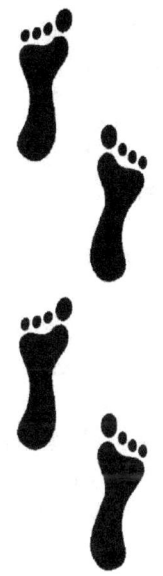

So now you've decided to at least start the journey and whether or not you elect to have WLS, the journey starts now.

For *most* people in *most* healthcare systems, there are classes and exercises, orientations, interviews and frustrations.

There are preparations and schedules to keep, appointments and time off of work to prepare for those appointments.

The journey is at times so all encompassing, the end goal becomes secondary.

When the pre-work gets larger than the end-result, perhaps a simple moment to refocus and reflect places "the journey" back into its proper perspective.

There have been instances when individuals were so driven by the preparation and/or classes mandatory to qualify for the surgery, they lost sight of the health aspects.

In fact, some have gotten so enthralled with the expectation of the outcome, focus was blurred, the weight loss did not occur and the WLS was cancelled.

There are a myriad of classes and support groups available for perspective WLS patients.

Some of the WLS preparation programs require one to lose a specific amount of weight before the surgery, which everyone knows is a journey all its own.

I was required to lose 10% which corresponds to 31 pounds, I was gung-ho and ended up losing about 48 pounds.

Some organizations even require a full psychiatric work up; each entity is a little different.

One thing is certain, whether you get to the operating table in seven weeks or seven years it is a journey.

I used a mind game to help myself reach my weight marks. I set several attainable milestones, or little baby goals I like to call them.

Unlike a race, a journey is an excursion, not to be attempted or embarked upon with haste.

Think of it as a journey/vacation to another country. You are all excited to begin the voyage, the anticipation is overwhelming.

Your bags are packed a month in advance, your passport picture is shiny and new, and you have a list of things to do once you arrive.

Oh my, by the time you go on the second walking tour, taken dozens of photos, posed at every tourist attraction, and slept in an uncomfortable bed in a strange hotel, the vacation/journey has lost its glamour.

By the time you're waiting to board the plane home you feel like intentionally knocking the other passengers in the head with your carry-on just to get on the plane and strapped in, in hopes of returning to the life you once complained was hopelessly mundane.

Patience is a virtue; however it happens to be the one most of us need to work on.

I know for sure, patience has never been my strong suit. I could always lose the weight with one of my quick, radical diets.

I wanted the weight off quickly!

But, each and every time the weight returned, once again forcing me to be patient and start again.

The decision and impending surgery will mirror this phase of your vacation, the anticipation will be great.

But the real challenge starts when you get home.

The surgery will seem like a daunting yet looming light at the end of a tunnel. Much like a vacation it will be anticipated with eagerness and excitement.

Your surgery date is just like a departure, you even have to pack for it!

Once you arrive at the hospital, just as the epiphany happens at the airport, reality sets in and you know this journey is all too real, no turning back.

The difference is, what you bring home is far more than a snow globe or t-shirt souvenir.

You bring home a new life! Ironically, WLS and vacation both cost a ton of money $$$.

You will walk through your front door with: an altered body, a new perspective, some pain, a new lifecycle, and soon a new body.

The souvenir you bring home from surgery will be with you forever.

It is uber important to grab hold of this one fact, sometimes the people around you will NOT understand your journey, but guess what. It aint (poor grammar intended) their journey, so they need not always understand it.

Perhaps, *your* journey is still in the packing or preparation phase?

Perhaps, you've decided against WLS and either want to do the diet/exercise route or need to take some time off.

Sorry to be a bit repetitive, but again I must say, IT'S OK!

When and if the time is right, you will know and act accordingly. WLS is not the only answer, nor the perfect answer.

WLS is simply a route and a tool one may choose to use.

"When you commit to the pursuit of personal growth, success cannot be far behind" –Charles Marshall

Your thoughts, questions, concerns, or notes:

Chapter 5 – The Surgery

"From every wound there is a scar, and every scar tells a story. A story that says I have survived. Turn your wounds into wisdom." - Unknown

As previously stated, the procedures and various WLSs available are as varied as the reasons to consider the surgery.

I selected Rouen-Y, a complete gastric bypass, which not only restricts the amount of food one can consume, but alters the body's ability to absorb what amount gets in.

I know my eating patterns and limitations, and I chose this procedure because of its restrictive and permanent qualities.

As previously stated, this book is not meant as a medical resource or even as a resource to inform you of what surgery is available.

I am not even trying to help you make your decision.

But I WANT YOU TO KNOW what I went through and some things that occur that medical professionals may not think is important.

Again, I want you to have someone or something to relate to, so you may know that you are NOT crazy.

Other people feel the same way and reacted the same way to this process.

I would have loved to have known that someone else out there was considering canceling the surgery the day of, or questioning their decision as the IV was being inserted.

More importantly, I would have loved if I'd known that I was not the only one thinking of all of the food I was NOT going to be able to eat for quite some time. Or maybe **never** would be able to eat for the rest of my life.

Oddly enough, a prevailing thought was of anger and frustration. I was angry that I had let myself go to the point that WLS was even necessary.

I was frustrated that my lack of will power had led me to this hospital.

More importantly, these thoughts in my head would have been easier to process had I had someone to talk to besides (my only option) spilling my guts in some open forum/group therapy sessions.

Or better yet, logging on and sharing with a bunch of faceless "real" nameless people who may or may not be telling the truth. Yet another reason why I am compelled to share my walk with you.

My surgery was scheduled for 12:30pm, so I had a lot of time to contemplate and think beforehand.

When I say a lot of time, I mean a lot of slow moving; seemingly never ending time, slow like cold syrup pouring out of a bottle, onto quickly cooling waffles.

By nature I am a morning person, and I am sure even those with the greatest faith do not sleep so soundly the day before surgery.

I digress; I made sure my home was clean as a whistle, my child cared for, and my overnight bag packed by 6:00am that morning.

In fact I went for a three mile walk before showering (walking had become a large part of my life, especially since my healthcare network required a 10% weight loss prior to approving the surgery).

After returning home I showered, sang, prayed and waited for my sister and niece to pick me up. Those hours ticked by at the speed of a 20lb turkey roasting on Thanksgiving afternoon with more than 20 hungry guests waiting (don't you love all of the food correlations).

I thought the time would never come. At last, my family drove up and as I opened the door we all erupted into laughter, for that is what my family does.

I instantly became the family's first WLS test subject.

What in the heck had I signed up for?

Once we arrived at the hospital things sped up, no really sped up.

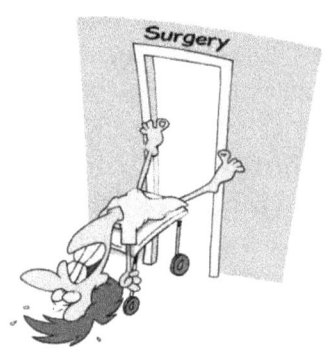

Before I realized it I'd registered, submitted my healthcare directive, paid my co-pay, and was getting poked and prodded.

Did I mention they weighed me?

Oh yes, I got weighed to ensure I was still at pre WLS goal.

Prayers... Lights... Nightie-night.... I am drifting to sleep.

"Nobody can go back and start a new beginning, but anyone can start today and make a new ending." –Maria Robinson

"Also let us remember that through any illness or difficult challenge, there is still much in life to be hopeful about and grateful for. We are infinitely more than our limitations or our afflictions." – Jeffrey R. Holland

Your thoughts, questions, concerns, or notes:

Your thoughts, questions, concerns, or notes:

Chapter 6 – What The @#$%^ Did I Just Do?

"New beginnings are often disguised as painful endings." –Lao Tzu

Now that you've had the surgery, it's time for your recovery.

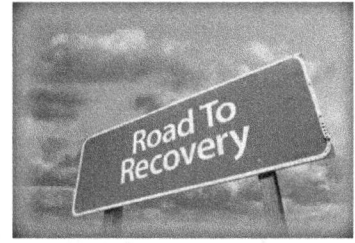

There are a number of things that go through one's mind immediately after waking from surgery.

I made it off of the table is the first thing I thought of after waking up from surgery.

Perhaps it was the second, I dunno but there was an overwhelming feeling of thank You Jesus, and I am alive.

I don't remember because the drugs for pain make everything nice and fuzzy.

However, I distinctly remember second guessing my decision to have surgery then immediately realizing it was too darn late to turn back!

My particular recovery wasn't too painful. I walked like a mad woman the weeks leading up to surgery, (I walked 3 miles the day of surgery, as previously stated).

Unbeknownst to me this all led to a surgery that went smoothly with little or no bleeding.

I walked because the pre op team urged me to do so, **but complied because** I wanted to maintain the pre surgery weight loss that was mandated by my physician so my WLS would not get cancelled.

All of this walking, although painful to my arthritic knees, helped me endure and recover well from WLS.

About 3 hours after surgery the nurse woke me up to take a walk.

The walk was surprisingly easy; I walked slowly with the IV pole and the nurse at first and picked up the pace after going a few feet.

I was given very small vials of broth and or water as well.

Again, the meds make one groggy so you don't have a full concept of the recovery until the next day.

I do recall feeling nauseous and somewhat bloated at the same time.

Before going to sleep for the evening I took another walk, this time without the nurse (but she was close by) and as I hobbled along with the IV pole again, the nausea rose and I began to vomit/burp/vomit but only clear liquid came out.

I was QUICKLY ushered back to my room to rest.

I would later find out that this was to prevent my sutures form tearing.

The following morning, I had the world's smallest breakfast.

I do not recall exactly what the meal consisted of, but I believe it was perhaps a portion of a scrambled egg.

Oddly enough I was totally full after eating just a portion. I knew then, my life would never be the same.

I was a girl who loved her bacon and egg sandwiches on sliced toasted bread with mayo or that tangy salad dressing, so being satisfied by a few bites was weird and very cool at the same time.

I was discharged from the hospital the following day with a ton of orders and suggestions from the team.

I went home and was amazed how my sister found every bump and crack in the road to hit on the way home in the car.

The good meds from the hospital were beginning to wear off, and I mean fast, LOL. Once at home, the adjustments began.

Once I climbed Mt. Everest. OK, so it just seemed that way.

Actually, once I climbed the flight of stairs to my bedroom and lay down in the bed I knew this would be something that would just take a little time and perseverance.

After all, I had had several surgeries (gall bladder, laparoscopic knee, etc.) not to mention a cesarean section birth, heck I could handle it.

In fact in one of the pre-WLS classes, the instructor admonished us not to run out and buy clothes too often, because undoubtedly we'd waste money and have to replace new garments with even newer ones.

I thought to myself, Now that's a problem I would LOVE to have, and didn't take it seriously.

Needless to say, the instructor was spot on, so take note people; garments with elastic and flowing outfits are your friends.

Garments without rigid seams shrink and grow with you.

Now if you are like me, the last thing you want to purchase to clothe your new slimmer body is clothing with elastic, no form, and extra material!

I mean let's be serious; showing off the new body is half the fun.

So if you subscribe to this mode of thought, budget accordingly and donate or swap clothes with other WLS recipients.

Approximately a month passed before others easily saw the weight loss, I began to learn what food and what amounts my body would accept and what did not work.

It was then when I realized, some of the warnings from the healthcare team were not etched in stone.

I began gingerly and INFREQUENTLY to test the boundaries. No, I was not supposed to!

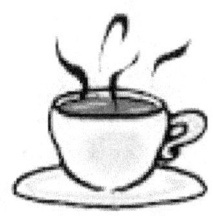

Coffee was one of the items that was strongly cautioned against.

I am not proud to say that to this day I still have 2 to 3 cups a day.

Some things are hard to surrender.

"Often people that criticize your life are usually the same people that don't know the price you paid to get where you are today." - myfavequotes.com

Your thoughts, questions, concerns, or notes:

Chapter 7 – The Mourning

"The secret of health for both mind and body is not to mourn for the past, worry about the future, or anticipate troubles, but to live in the present moment wisely and earnestly." –Buddha

"Blessed are those who mourn, for they shall be comforted." –Matthew 5:4

Yes, yes it is time to gripe!

A time to mourn, and time to complain.

Let the bitterness begin, if only for a season.

So I began to think to myself (because I was the only person who I could relate to initially), hey this is not so fair.

So let me get this right; I can't eat popcorn with extra butter at the movies, I can't drink insane amounts of my specialty coffee, I can't drink mojitos into the wee hours of the morning on a night out with the girls, I can't indulge on Thanksgiving like everyone else and pass out early in bed.

I can't watch the Food Network all night then make all the gooey gushy things I see and eat them! I can't order too much fried chicken from Popeye's and regret it the next day?

I can't read a book when I am lonely and eat caramel cake to celebrate each chapter's end?

What the heck? This aint cool at all!

Gripe #2! Why is Tina, my coworker, the biggest junk food junkie known to man and skinny as a rail?

Why are most of the women on the food channels making all of this stuff yet look like runway models?

This crap is so not fair. Lastly, why do I have to go through this drastic and life altering process to get healthy, feel better, and look good?

I slowly realized girlfriend... life is not always fair, get over it and move on.

I recalled a conversation my mother had with my aunt when I was a child (yes, I was eavesdropping). My mother suffered from severe emphysema for many years and was bed ridden.

My aunt got into bed with her on a visit, the conversation waxed deep and I snooped even deeper.

My mom asked my aunt, why her? What had she done to deserve this fate, this illness?

My aunt very calmly told my mom, "Honey, they crucified Jesus and He didn't do anything but go around healing and saving." Sometimes we endure things that aren't fair, but others endure more.

At that moment I knew the ability to put things in their proper perspective would help me for the rest of my life.

As I remembered all I had been through to get to this point, and what the alternatives may have been, I sat back, dried my tears, and put it all into perspective.

I knew that whether it was genetics, environment, emotion, or just plain old over indulging that put me in this place, it did not define me. I was bigger and better and more blessed than this blue funk.

No matter how I got here, I thought to myself; *Shut Up! Get Over It! And do what is needed to be done to Fix It!*

And for goodness sakes, put some make up on and comb your hair (sorry gentlemen, I got nothin' for you this paragraph).

And by all means friends (yeah, you are my friend now), know that it is ok to occasionally throw away food.

Of course we all desire to exercise wisdom when ordering, preparing, or purchasing food.

However (don't you love all of my "however statements"), sometimes leaving food on your plate, in your fridge, and at the restaurant will be necessary to stave off illness, not to mention weight gain (see latter chapters).

Listen, waste is not a good thing, nor do I encourage it.

But guess what, the last two bites of food can NOT be molecularly transported to hungry children across the world.

Go donate, volunteer, or adopt to stave off your guilt. I admonish you, discard or give away the rest of your food once your stomach says no.

When mourning your old relationship with food, think of it in this way.

Remember when your relationship ended with him or her and you reminisced about the good times you had?

You'd sit back and remember when he took you to that awesome movie and you kissed for the first time or she baked you a cake for your birthday and it was the first time a girl had done something so thoughtful for you.

Now, you call your best friend and she reminds you that the movie date wasn't all that great because you had to pay for his ticket and you went on the bus because his car broke down.

Or for you guys, your bro called you to console you, and reminded you that you got food poisoning from the cake she baked and there are still stains in the carpet from when her dog knocked it over.

Well food memories are like that, in retrospect they seem like they were the best eats of your life.

But the trouble they cause in the end simply take away the fondness.

Take the power from the popover, the glam from the grilled cheese, take the mmmm from the mint chip ice cream.

At its core, food is sustenance, energy, fuel.

Sustenance we enjoy and crave, but sustenance still.

We have the ability to build fond memories based on the relationships we built while getting ice cream.

But the relationships and memories are not created because of the food, but rather in spite of.

"The truth is, unless you let go, unless you forgive yourself, unless you forgive the situation, unless you realize that the situation is over, you cannot move forward." – Steve Maraboli

Your thoughts, questions, concerns, or notes:

Chapter 8 – The Reactions

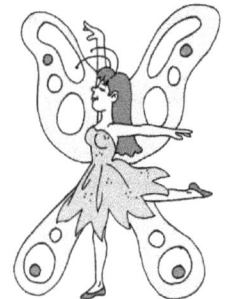

"When she transformed into a butterfly, the caterpillars spoke not of her beauty, but of her weirdness. They wanted her to change back into what she always had been. But she had wings." –Dean Jackson

People are going to say, "You've changed since you've had that surgery."

Every single WLS patient I have ever spoken with has encountered this proclamation.

Not everyone means it in a negative manner, and some do.

But, more than likely as your shape changes, your life and relationships will follow suit.

Know this. *When someone says, "You've changed," it simply means you've stopped living your life their way.*" –Unknown

And guess what, if a person is not growing and changing, chances are they are dying.

So perhaps you are changing a bit, pray and watch that it is for the better and not the worse.

You're darned if you do and darned if you don't, that's how it feels at times.

If people know that you are considering WLS and you do not proceed, people are going to think you are weak.

Some will say if you don't have the will power to lose the weight, at least have the guts to get on the operating table.

For those who react unfavorably, WHO CARES!

Get ready! People are going to treat you differently, I dare say like crap at times.

Find comfort in knowing that you cannot change the people around you, but you can change the people you select to be around. You can change **your** reactions to **their** words.

So, exercise your options with **love** and **wisdom**.

I was the president and treasurer of the *"People Pleasing Club."*

I was no angel, but I was the one who relinquished my position in a discussion or gave up the seat in a crowded room.

If there was a task to be done, or a person to please, I volunteered. If there was a family issue to moderate, I played referee.

There are a multitude of reasons why I always took a back seat, and made sure everyone else was happy.

My size? My upbringing? My birth order?

Who knows, but once I started to take care of me and drop the weight I unconsciously dropped some of the need to please people.

When I evolved, it was perceived as me becoming a bitch because I thought I was "cute and thin," they said.....

Oh well. Perception is defined in part as: *a way of regarding, understanding, or interpreting something; a mental impression.*

And guess what, it is all relative and is dependent upon each person's contextual life experiences. So, if you are seen as changing...

OK.... Do a self-check; make sure your integrity did not diminish, along with your weight.

This is the crux of this chapter; people in general are not fans of change.

Do not allow people to make more withdrawals than deposits in your life!

Do not constantly entertain and give ear to the naysayers and negative noise.

People said to me on more than one occasion, you are so pretty now.

What later rang in my mind was the belief that I had always been beautiful.

Not in the aesthetic or superficial arrogant way, but in in the eyes of GOD and family kind of way.

Just because I made a choice to become healthier and stronger, that choice did not make me or you more beautiful, you may be more pleasing in THEIR eyes, but you were always that way.

I knew God had made me beautiful from the beginning, I just did not realize it.

Here are some helpful mottos, quips, and quotes for this time in your life.

"New beginnings are often disguised as painful endings." – Lao Tzu

"Don't waste words on people who deserve your silence. Sometimes the most powerful thing you can say is nothing at all." - Mandy Hale

"Respect yourself enough to walk away from anything that no longer serves you, grows you, or makes you happy." – Unknown

"Perfection is not attainable, but if we chase perfection we can catch excellence." –Vince Lombardi.

What Vince did not say is, *God has given us an awesome example of excellence, all we have to do is follow His lead.*

Your thoughts, questions, concerns, or notes:

Chapter 9 – Processing The Anger

"Anger is an acid that can do more harm to the vessel in which it is stored than to anything on which it is poured." –Mark Twain

"Hey Slim!" "What's up skinny Minnie?" "Hey baby, what's your name?"

*"Girl, your clothes look really cute, **now**!" "Eh you, can I holla at you a minute, men have started to knock down your door, **hunh**?"*

That receptionist has been dropping off your office supplies for years, but now she smiles at you and calls you mister.

Oh the lovely comments never cease.

And these are just the comments from the people we know.

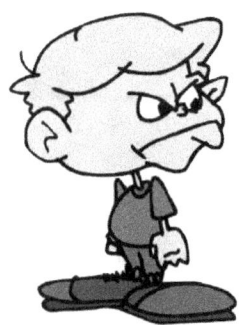

We won't attempt to address comments from passersby that we may have encountered at work or the library... but we were never noticed by them before!

What gives people the unmitigated gall, or permission to comment openly and freely about our private journey?

Through the annals of time, weight has been the one subject that many people feel comfortable discussing or asking questions about publically to and about someone.

Even if the comment was clearly not solicited.

Don't believe me? Try these comments on for size.

Have you ever seen someone approached by a cursory friend and associate, and ask them, *"Hey, I've noticed you lie to a lot of people, why do you do that so often?"* or *"I noticed you drank two more glasses of wine than the rest of us, are you an alcoholic?"* or *what about, "I see you walk your dog with that same person daily, and your socks have rainbows on them, are you gay?"*

Nope, it is likely those comments and questions may never be uttered. Such phrases are considered rude or passé. Conversely, when it comes to the subject of weight, social protocol is often ignored.

Here's a prime example. There was a sales associate at a chain clothing store I frequented. This sales person, a well groomed, size 10 woman in her early 60s knew my face from my shopping trips, but not my name.

She confidently and unashamedly asked me, *"What did you do to lose all of that weight? You are much prettier now, what size is that in your hand? Did you have that surgery?"*

"You can stop losing the weight now, because you don't want to look to gaunt."

People.... It is probably gonna happen to you so brace yourself and breathe.

The pinnacle of my anger surfaced due to an incident with another woman, not a man, ironically enough.

This woman often was my lunch partner at work, with whom I spent many breaks and lunches.

I had lost weight. One day upon returning from a lunch (at which I am certain I ate a much smaller portion than she did), she had to park in a snug parking space. After gingerly exiting her vehicle, and making certain not to scratch either car (as always), she said "I can park in those spaces now because I know when you get out you won't bang the car anymore."

In my head I thought, What the !@#$? I never banged any car, even at my top weight! But aloud I said nothing because I was too taken aback by the comment.

That comment confirmed a long suspected suspicion of mine, people think fat people are less than ____, you fill in the blank.

I don't know about you, but this is how I feel about it, and I will be totally honest about this (ouch).

I was mad! Mad at the cat calls from men that came with more abundance AFTER the weight loss.

Mad at the people making unwarranted and unwanted comments about my weight (before, during, or after).

Mad at the old ladies at church not using kind words to inquire about my journey, mad at everyone and everything. WHEEHW... that felt good to admit.

I was ticked off, do you understand. But then, I realized that the anger tainted the journey.

The anger gave the purveyors of negativity the last hurrah, and that belonged exclusively to me.

This is a Quote Frenzy Alert!!! To sum it up, the way my daughter would phrase it;

"Haters are going to hate on you" ...but find comfort knowing that haters don't really hate you. In fact, they hate themselves because you are a reflection of what they want to be.

Give the anger the smallest most transient place in your journey, it deserves nothing more.

Watch your words when processing the anger, "Always, remember pain makes people change. So don't hurt them, if you don't want them to change." -Unknown

"Throughout life people will make you mad, disrespect you and treat you bad. Let GOD deal with the things they do, because hate in your heart will consume you too." –Will Smith

"Life becomes easier when you learn to accept an apology you never got" –Robert Brault

Your thoughts, questions, concerns, or notes:

Chapter 10 –The Loss

Yes, mourning and loss are different.

"There is sacredness in tears; they are not the mark of weakness, but of power. They speak more eloquently than ten thousand tongues. They are the messengers of overwhelming grief, of deep contrition, and of unspeakable love." – Washington Irving

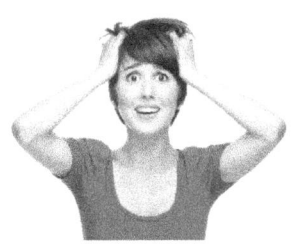

Loss of appetite, loss of hair, loss of taught skin, loss of food related satisfaction, loss of energy, loss of clothing, loss of shoe size, loss of boobage (aka cleavage/décolletage), loss of sleep, loss of being comfortable in all your old skin, loss of friends, loss of warmth (post WLS most patients have temperature regulating issues- hello, you've in essence been wearing a coat for years), and finally loss of pounds.

Everything that is lost does not necessarily need to be found.

Society would have you to minimize these losses after WLS.

Society asks that we solely concentrate on all that you have apparently gained such as: freedom from excess weight and related illness.

Freedom from medication. Freedom to wear more clothes (or less☺), freedom to be slimmer. However, I beg to differ.

Whenever a person loses something or someone which has been a significant part of their lives, my goodness it is going to be missed.

You may not feel comfortable admitting it, but absence of "old self" is going to take time and effort to get accustomed to.

Have you ever lost something you could not live without, but only after an exhaustive search do you come to the realization that continued energy looking for it just isn't worth it?

An analogy I love to use is the house slipper analogy.

Many of us at one point in our lives have possessed a favorite article of clothing, personal item, or in my case house slippers.

Now, my pair of house slippers had definitely seen better days; they were at least 4 years old, unevenly worn down, thread bare, discolored, and barely intact.

However, I loved, loved, loved those slippers.

These slippers were: dependable and predictable in fit, familiar.

One day the slippers disappeared, personally I think my ex-boyfriend threw them out (he didn't care for them).

Guess what happened, within days, I not only stopped searching for those slippers, but I no longer missed them.

Enough said!

There is no need to belabor this subject, so let's tie up this loss stuff and move on!

NO, I am not minimizing loss, just minimizing how much of your existence it should occupy.

"Life begins, at the end of your comfort zone." – Unknown

"Trust in the Lord with all your heart, and lean not on your own understanding; in all your ways acknowledge Him, and He will direct your paths." Proverbs 3:5-6

Your thoughts, questions, concerns, or notes:

Chapter 11 – The Plateau

"Be proud of yourself NOW, not when you've reached your goal. A plateau is nothing more than a landing which allows you time to catch your breath so you can continue to climb." -Unknown

For once, do something for you.

Yes, you may desire to lose weight to be able to play with your children or make sure you are even around *for* them. Perhaps you want to lose weight for medical or emotional reasons or want to attract a spouse.

But, this begins and ends with YOU. So, you are the one who has to contend with this plateau.

Know this. A plateau is simply that, a resting place and somewhere and sometime to regroup.

What would one normally do on a plateau in the physical realm?

He or she would regroup, assess what is ahead, what has been left behind and decide on a plan of attack to get to the next level.

Well, that is what this plateau is affording you, a time to regroup.

This time of introspection and reflection applies if you HAVE OR HAVE NOT decided to proceed on the WLS journey.

A plateau is a useful tool and not an enemy, this mode of thought applies to life and is especially spot-on if you are on a journey of wellness.

Some may hit plateaus trying to reach goal weight before surgery, or even after WLS.

This is my advice, simply do some reading, researching, or even reach out to healthcare professionals and nutrition experts.

You would be amazed how helpful a fresh eye, and new perspective, may be.

A neutral and unbiased assessment of your current eating and exercise program may identify modifications that need to occur.

Believe it or not, a fresh angle on a subject often identifies issues that were simply invisible to the one too close to the matter.

If you've ever been a "certified dieter" (sounds so much more professional when stated that way eh?) like myself, you know there are times when no matter what you do or how strictly you adhere to your program the weight loss stalls.

When the plateau hits, the usual reaction is one of frustration, anger, or defeat.

None of those emotions are going to help you reach the next level, only P's can do that.

P's are: Patience, Perseverance, Prayer, Planning, and Positivity.

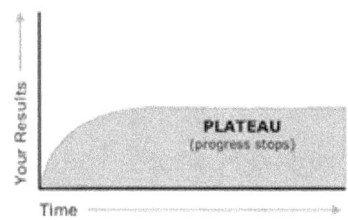

I hit two plateaus in my journey, the first quite early on, approximately six months after WLS.

After having the gastric bypass I lost weight extremely quickly.

I mean, it seemed as though each day I would have to adjust my clothing to account for the rapid weight loss.

But that did not last long! After about six months, I realized that the drastic weight loss had slowed to a crawl. In fact I noticed, I hadn't met my post WLS goal weight yet, so what is going on?

I went to a regular post-op check-up with the surgeon and realized that the slowed weight loss was common, but there were a few rules I had not adhered to that also lent to the stall.

I implemented those minute but crucial changes and soon was back on track.

The second plateau was five years post WLS, about 2012. I simply got comfortable being 170 pounds with little effort.

For me, 170 allowed me the moderately pain -ree mobility and the fashion latitude I was comfortable with, I am just being honest.

For my 5'1" frame, I was still too heavy by medical standards, but honestly I was ok with it.

The exercise waned, my commute increased, the knees began to hurt a bit more, and I began to stretch the core "rules for life" bit by bit and I even began to drink ginger ale in copious amounts.

I justified the carbonated beverage consumption by telling myself that it was helping my occasional upset stomach.

But really, I wanted some sweet fizz. Hence, the weight stalled, then ever so gradually began an upward swing (but that is another chapter).

What did I do to climb to the next level, you may ask? I got back on track and reinstituted the original post WLS diet.

Some of the weight began to drop back off, but I am still on this journey. For me walking and water consumption is key, and eating at night is the enemy.

As the older ladies at church would say, God aint through with me yet. I continue to live a healthier live, and fight the good fight.

"Strength shows, not only in the ability to persist, but the ability to start over." –Unknown

Chapter 12 – The Addiction Substitute

> *"It is impossible to understand addiction without asking what relief the addict finds or hopes to find, in the drug or addictive behavior."* -Gabor Mate

What's your addiction?

I refuse to call it anything else like habit, bliss, dependency issue. I do not sugar coat much.

Is your addiction shopping, dating, social media-ing, exercising, **sex**ing, wine-ing, and whining, medicating, eating, churching, volunteering, etc?

Be honest, you already know that something may not be right friend. For most, food filled some kind of void, provided some sort of pleasure... release... and helped those endorphins flow.

So now that the food (in its old form) is gone, something or someone is likely to take its place.

I will be the first to admit, I considered the addiction classes mandated by my health care provider (before they would give the WLS green light) WORTHLESS and a waste of time!

Little did I know, I would rely heavily on the tools I learned in class to help me on my journey.

I was the consummate pessimist... read carefully now. *"I am not fat because I am eating to satisfy some longing or deep rooted unresolved issue. I am eating because I am hungry dammit."* < That was me 100%>

What I came to realize is, it doesn't matter if one *believes* that the food issue is born of a deep conflict or has a root cause.

The fact is, there is probably a food issue and/or addiction. Period.

So the food issue must be addressed, because whatever filled the void, or satiated-experience food provided, will need to be replaced by something.

Let's hope it is a good something.

Friend, because we are humans and not androids, we naturally enjoy endorphins.

When endorphins are released, it is because we participated in an activity which brings *temporary* pleasure.

Thus we desire to recreate or re-enact that thing which released that well feeling or endorphin rich moment.

We as humans want and desire to feel good, so we chase after the feeling, whether knowingly or blissfully unaware.

For some, they replace the food with exercise. For some it is dating.

It may appear harmless, and even beneficial.

No matter what it is, anything that is in excess or too consuming should be addressed and acknowledged.

Endorphins are: any group of hormones secreted within the brain and nervous system and having a number of physiological functions.

They are peptides that activate the body's opiate receptors, causing an analgesic effect.

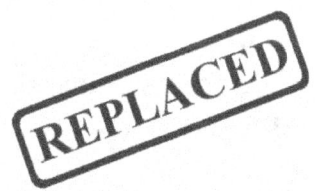

In short they make you feel good. Now, this is where many folk (me too) get off track.

When the food crutch is gone, and you have this new body and new outlook, the options of what to replace the food with are endless.

I mean, it is as if a new world has opened up to you, especially if you were a wall flower such as myself.

Again, some addictions, like volunteering or working out can be good.

However, in most instances, they do not release the same feeling of wellness and joy provided by some of the more negative addictions.

I will be honest. Initially I would have one glass of red wine before or after dinner on occasion.

I quickly saw that becoming one glass a night, then two.

When (transparent to me) the consumption got out of hand, God did something awesome, my stomach began to get quite upset whenever wine was consumed. Incidentally, wine is on most healthcare providers Do Not Ingest list, post WLS.

Something that could have been a real issue was resolved for me, that spontaneous biological change is what I call **grace and favor**.

My second addiction challenge came in the form of pain medication.

The primary reason I chose WLS was to increase my mobility.

My knees were shot to heck! Bone on bone, advanced arthritis in both.

At the age of 36 I had to spend at least one day a week in bed resting my knees and to reduce swelling.

I was a single working mother of a 13 year old girl.

My life had to change; I was too young for such a life, I believed.

Because my overall health was quite good, my doctor strongly suggested WLS.

He said my life would change drastically for the better, and I would be doing myself and my daughter a disservice if I did not consider it.

My doctor's words were a huge catalyst for me considering WLS.

I thought of myself as selfish if I didn't do everything in power to give my daughter the best mother possible.

Needless to say after WLS, a hysterectomy, several laparoscopic knee procedures, and later one total knee replacement, pain mediation was a well-integrated part of my life.

In fact, it was too much a part of my life.

I'd wake up with one or two pain pills to get enough relief to get going, and go to sleep with the same.

Perhaps I would have some pain pills in the middle of the day too, if I deemed them necessary.

Please realize that post WLS, food is not the only thing our bodies process differently.
My tolerance for pain and pain medication was extremely high.

What offered someone pain relief did not necessarily affect me the same way.

I am NOT making excuses, only sharing my walk.

It was not easy, but through prayer and persistence, pain mediation had to be put in its place as a tool, and not a rule.

So now, what's my issue?

I tend to be the "I will do it, run there for you, clean up after the party, organize the soiree, chauffeur the teens, write that resume..." kind of person.

At times, I am so busy with the business of being helpful, I forget my own limitations and lend myself to be leaned on or used up.

Sounds a lot like chapter six right?

I am still finding my happy place, my healthy addiction. I will never give up the fight for a life of balance.
We can, and will, win this race friend.

We must take the WLS journey without gaining another piece of baggage (literal or physical), not another pound!

First, there must be acknowledgment. If something other than food has taken hold and occupies a space that food used to, admit it.

We all know that there are some things that make you feel good, that are not good for you. It's ok to ask for help. Please, ask for help.

"Life is a balance of holding on and letting go" - *Rumi*

Your thoughts, questions, concerns, or notes:

Chapter 11 – The Fear of Regaining The Weight

"When your past calls don't answer. It has nothing new to say" – Anonymous

F-E-A-R has two meanings: Forget everything and run OR Face everything and rise. The choice is yours" – Zig Ziglar

The F-A-C-T (the implication) Facing the actual cause truthfully: regaining the weight is possible.

What may cause fear and anxiety for a post WLS patient? One simple thought; we will wake up one day and realize the weight has returned.

It does not matter if the boomerang weight regain happened gradually or quickly, but the fear of the return weight is all too real.

The fear of weight gain is real and I feel it every single day.

Not the kind of crippling, oppressing fear but a healthy one that encourages me to employ and stick to the tried and true rules for success that most healthcare providers offer.

This kind of fear is based in respect, similar to the fear of God and the fear based in respect for His Word and Will.

A healthy, not hindering fear is what I am experiencing now. This fear makes me make better choices, and avoid bad ones.

So here I am almost eight years post WLS (yeah I've been writing this book for several years –she hangs head in shame) and let me tell you, the last 2 years nothing has haunted me more than facing the fact of possible weight regain.

(WARNING, here I go with another quote!)

"You're not the same individual you were a year ago, a month ago, or a week ago. You're always growing. Experiences don't stop. That's life." - Osiris

Allow me to be totally honest here, for me my food challenge was intertwined with love.

I was dating my now husband. My slightly rotund, loves to take me out to eat husband.

And guess what, stuff changes.

You can know in your heart, psyche, intellect, and will that something should be off limits, but gosh darn it when your honey says, "please take a bite, taste this, try this sauce," (at least in my case) those small voices take a dumb vacation.

So yes, there was some moderate weight gain, and I am still **fighting the good fight** as many gospel ministers say.

The fact is, weight return is real but should not consume you or negate the awesomeness of your courage and growth gained on the WLS journey.

For certain the medical community has volumes of data and cautions about return weight post WLS.

Of course, after the plateau many experience moderate to significant weight gain.

Our bodies are smart machines, and often times they find an internal middle ground that ensures it operates optimally.

I am almost in my sweet spot, after my marriage weight gain I am finally finding that moderate exercise and going back to the basics is what will work best for me.

As stated earlier, of course there will be those people!!

What people you may ask? Those people, who were just watching and waiting (some wishing and hoping) your weight would return.

I have certainly witnessed both sides of the spectrum, those who have WLS and stay at goal weight long term and some who shortly after, regain the weight and experience little or no long term success.

I am in the middle, I am no longer 310 pounds, I am no longer a size 9 (my lowest weight), but I am a fluffy size 14. I am ok with that, as long as my health is solid and my path sure.

So pay attention to this little nugget of truth, a setback or a fear of one, does now define you!

Sometimes success is only attained after several attempts and failures.

I saw this quote once and it brought me much comfort, the late Nelson Mandela said, *"I learned that courage was not the absence of fear, but the triumph over it. The brave man is not he who does not feel afraid, but he who conquers that fear."*

Lastly, after complaining to my niece about having to repeat steps in my weight loss journey, she very calmly said: "genuine success, for some, may require multiple attempts."

Be confidant and know, although your process may be slower than others, it is better to learn to close a door quietly and firmly rather than swiftly and loudly...only for it to bounce back open again!

Life is like a camera, just focus on what's important and capture the good times. Develop from the negatives and if things don't work out, just take another shot.

Your thoughts, questions, concerns, or notes:

Your thoughts, questions, concerns, or notes:

Chapter 12 – The Faith in Yourself, Your Decisions, and in God

"Stress makes you believe that everything has to happen right now. Faith reassures you that everything will happen in God's timing!" - Unknown

"Cast your burden on the Lord and He will sustain you, He will never permit the righteous to be moved." –Psalm 55:22

Here are twelve tips to help you on your faith journey.

For me this began and ended with my Christian Faith. God is truly the finest example of being faithful.

For you, faith may come from a different place... but know that faith is key to your resolve and confidence in knowing ... this too shall pass. You can accomplish that which you set your mind to, even if setbacks occur and paths change.

Always ensure that your faith is bigger than your fear.

But always know, faith is a verb in my book.

Faith is an action term and gives as good as it gets. So work your faith and let it work for you.

"Action" faith is based in real conversation and self-talk, for example:

1. Have faith that if it doesn't feel right, it probably is not right for you.
2. Say what is on your mind, in a respectful tone. Have faith that getting it out will make you feel better, because there is more room out than in.
3. Have faith that everyone may not be pleased with your words or actions.
4. Have faith that no one is perfect, not even you.
5. Have faith you can and will endure through it all.
6. Have faith that Yes is ok to say.
7. Have faith that No is ok to say.
8. Have faith that it is ok not to have complete closure about every doggone thing.
9. Have faith in knowing that you are loved!
10. Have faith that you are but flesh and blood, not making excuses but acknowledging the fallibly.
11. Have faith in your beauty, YES YOU ARE BEAUTIFUL.
12. Have faith that you can overcome obstacles.

*** FAITH = Forward All Issues to Heaven ***

"Learn to trust that still small voice you often stifle. It is **that** voice which reminds you of the truth your mind has yet to accept." -Me

Your thoughts, questions, concerns, or notes:

Your thoughts, questions, concerns, or notes:

Your Chapter – Make Peace with Your Decision

"Peace is the result of retraining your mind to process life as it is, rather than as you think it should be." –Wayne W. Dyer

Spoiler Alert! Ok, not to spoil the ending for you, but I just so happen to know the ending to your story.

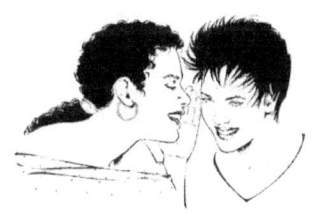

Come close, closer, now listen: **Everything is going to work out**.

Now that I've said it, the secret is out.

You've made it to the end of the book, and more importantly to a milestone on your journey.

Take a breath, it's going to be OK.

If you've made the decision to not have WLS, be ok with it.

If you have made the decision TO have WLS, that is ok too.

OWN your decision and rest in the knowledge that all is well if you are well.

You are the editor of your book, and God is the author.

He has given us unrestricted editing privileges that may or may not make the book a best seller but one thing is for sure my friend, you are not alone.

"Everything will be ok in the end, and if it is not ok, it's not the end." -Unknown

Your thoughts, questions, concerns, or notes:

Your Beginning – Never the End!

Here's to the rest of your life. I wish you peace, blessings, health, and happiness.

"Give it to GOD, and go to sleep."

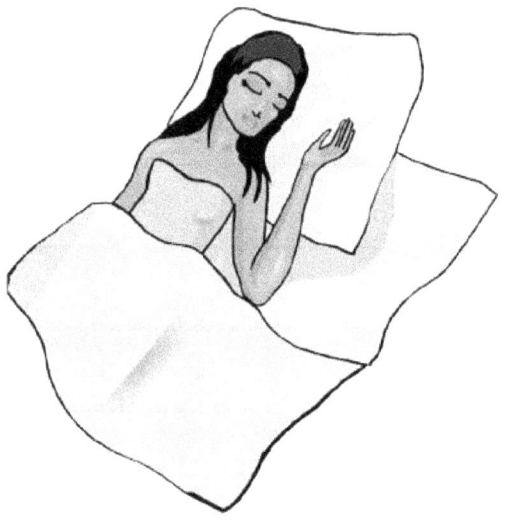

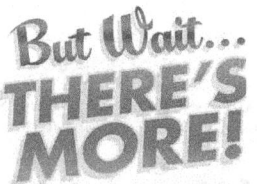 I wrote this book for both you and me, so I'd love to have your thoughts, experiences, feedback and comments.

Please go to my web site listed below.

You'll find a BLOG where you can give me your inputs, feedback, and experiences.

Who knows, I might just write another book and need to ask you for your experiences.

www.ArlandasInsights.com

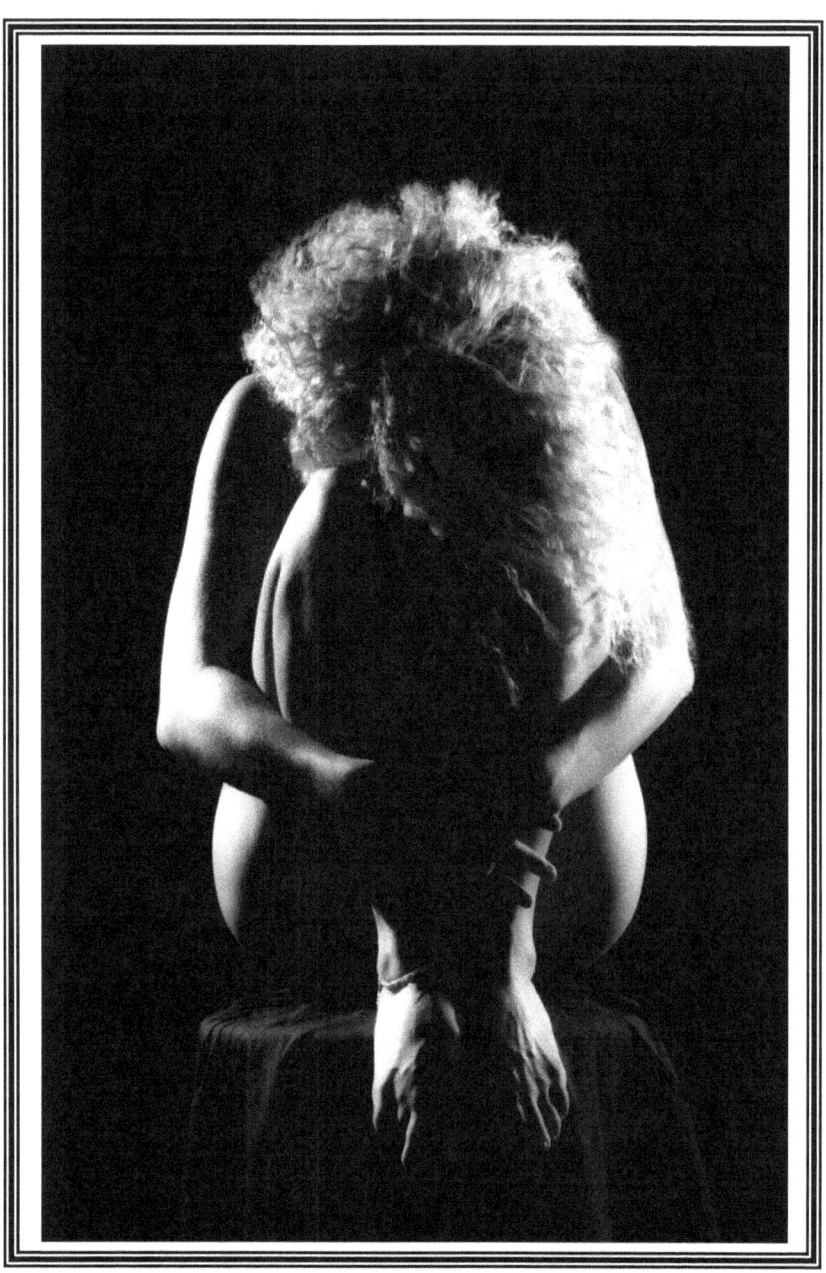

www.ingramcontent.com/pod-product-compliance
Lightning Source LLC
Chambersburg PA
CBHW072039190526
45165CB00018B/1184